Health Benefits of Probiotics

Healthy Living Series

M. Usman

Mendon Cottage Books

JD-Biz Publishing

All Rights Reserved.

No part of this publication may be reproduced in any form or by any means, including scanning, photocopying, or otherwise without prior written permission from JD-Biz Corp Copyright © 2014

All Images Licensed by Fotolia and 123RF.

Disclaimer

The information is this book is provided for informational purposes only. It is not intended to be used and medical advice or a substitute for proper medical treatment by a qualified health care provider. The information is believed to be accurate as presented based on research by the author.

The contents have not been evaluated by the U.S. Food and Drug Administration or any other Government or Health Organization and the contents in this book are not to be used to treat cure or prevent disease.

The author or publisher is not responsible for the use or safety of any diet, procedure or treatment mentioned in this book. The author or publisher is not responsible for errors or omissions that may exist.

Warning

The Book is for informational purposes only and before taking on any diet, treatment or medical procedure, it is recommended to consult with your primary health care provider.

Check out some of the other Healthy Gardening Series books at Amazon.com

Gardening Series on Amazon

Check out some of the other Health Learning Series books at Amazon.com

Health Learning Series on Amazon

Table of Contents

Getting Started

Chapter # 1: Intro

Bacteria are notoriously known for causing and spreading various diseases in the body, so the whole idea of consuming a few billion of them a day for the goodness of one's health may seem, both figuratively and literally, hard to swallow! But in the last decade there has been an increasing amount of positive evidence that suggests that many of these bacteria in foods and supplements can actually cure illnesses and eliminate their underlying causes. These "good" bacteria are known as probiotics and are the new big thing in the scientific community.

The word "probiotics" is a composite of the Greek words, "pro" and "biotic". The word "pro" means to amplify promotion while "biotic" means life, therefore, combine the two words and you get something along the lines of "to promote life". This word-definition fits the description to quite a large extent; the World Health Origination defines probiotics as any live microorganism that provides a health benefit when consumed. Similar descriptions have been provided by other medical research bodies. For most people who are familiar with the word, the mention of probiotics brings up images of yogurt and other fermented food items, but it must be noted that probiotics are not just found in yogurt but can be actively cultured. Nowadays, probiotics are commonly available in supplements in the form of capsules, liquids or in chewable form; a number of strains are sold in the market but the most popular ones are Lactobacillus and Bifidobacteria. Don't be horrified by their gigantic names as none of your doubts and queries will go unresolved.

Chapter # 2: Diving in Deeper

Our digestive system is home to what we can call good bacteria and bad bacteria; it is absolutely necessary for optimum health that our body maintains the correct balance between these good bacteria and bad bacteria. External factors like medications, diseases and change in diet can disturb this balance. Sometimes the body is able to relapse on its own while sometimes it can't. Read on further and find out the reasons behind ailments caused by an upset in this balance.

Probiotics are believed to play a very important role in regulating intestinal functions, like digestion, by a system known as intestinal microflora. This microflora is a health mechanism that positively influences the normal functional growth of the intestinal system.

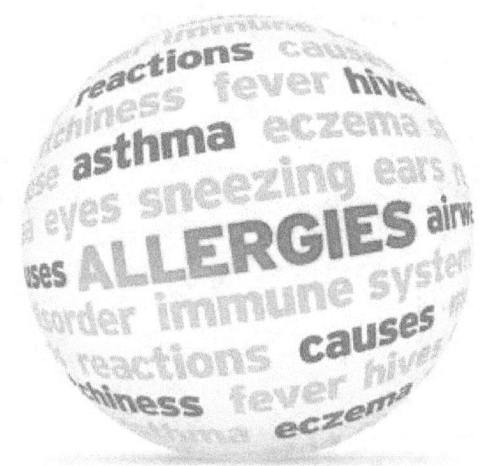

What is the gut? Many of us have heard the term "gut feeling" which is a sense towards something without exactly knowing the reason behind it. Many people are also known to experience their emotions in their stomach but no one knows why. Recently, scientists have discovered a whole network of neurons, lined up in our gut, with the network being so extensive that the nickname "second brain" was given to it. This gut brain might not have good thinking skills, but it does play an elementary part in communicating with our brain and spotting diseases within the tract. Technically speaking, the lining of neurons in the gastrointestinal tract forms the *enteric* nervous system. Its role is to manage every aspect of digestion in all the organs within the tract including colon, small intestine, esophagus and stomach. It uses over a hundred million neurons and other chemical mechanisms that are found in the "real" brain. Within this gastrointestinal tract, there is the microflora which encompasses over 400 bacterial species, many of which are classified as probiotics. The intestinal microflora not only aids in digestion but also helps synthesize vitamins and nutrients, support the development of the gut, and enhance the immune system. All of this explains why it is absolutely necessary for the body to be in possession of probiotics.

Moreover, self-dosing one's self with these good bacteria isn't as outlandish as it might sound; an estimated 100 trillion microorganisms belonging from over 500 different cultures inhabit a healthy bowel.

Probiotics are known to work in the following areas:

1. Digestive Health
2. Urinary Health
3. Allergies
4. Women's Health
5. Immunity
6. Obesity

The body begins to reap the benefits provided by probiotics right from one's birth; during a delivery through the birth canal, a newborn picks up a number of bacteria from his/her mother and thereby develops immunity to many diseases. Unfortunately, these bacteria are not transferred during a cesarean birth and this has been the reason behind many infants picking up allergies resulting in less than normal level of immunity and lower levels of gut flora.

It has been stated earlier that a fine balance between good and bad bacteria is essential to ensure a healthy digestive tract. A fit digestive tract effectively filters out, as well as, eliminates any harmful element in the body such as toxins, bad bacteria, chemicals and other waste materials, while on the good side, it takes in the good stuff for the body, absorbs it and helps in its delivery to the cell in need. The principle is not to eliminate every single bad bacterium, but to produce a balanced environment, because as soon as the balance tips off, ailments such as muscle pain, diarrhea, fatigue and urinary tract infections follow.

Another way in which probiotics help the body make a preemptive strike on several diseases is by boosting up the immune system. Many scientists acclaim this role and consider it the most important one when it comes to probiotics. The immune system is the first line of defense against germs and all the hazardous risks they carry. When the immune system fails to function properly, the body suffers from autoimmune disorders and allergic reactions like Crohn's disease, rheumatoid arthritis and ulcerative colitis. Furthermore, the body can get infections like diarrhea and also skin ones. Probiotics make sure that the balance remains in the favor of the body and therefore prevents these ailments.

Chapter # 3: Types of Probiotics

Up until the 60s, the microflora in the gut was thought to be caused by bacteria, namely clostridia, enterococci, lactobacilli and Escherichia coli, but since then a number of new innovative techniques have been able to show that there are actually many more varieties of bacteria at work in the gut. There are several different kinds of probiotics, with each one being identified by its species, strain level, and genus. The following are some of the most commonly known bacteria along with their health benefits:

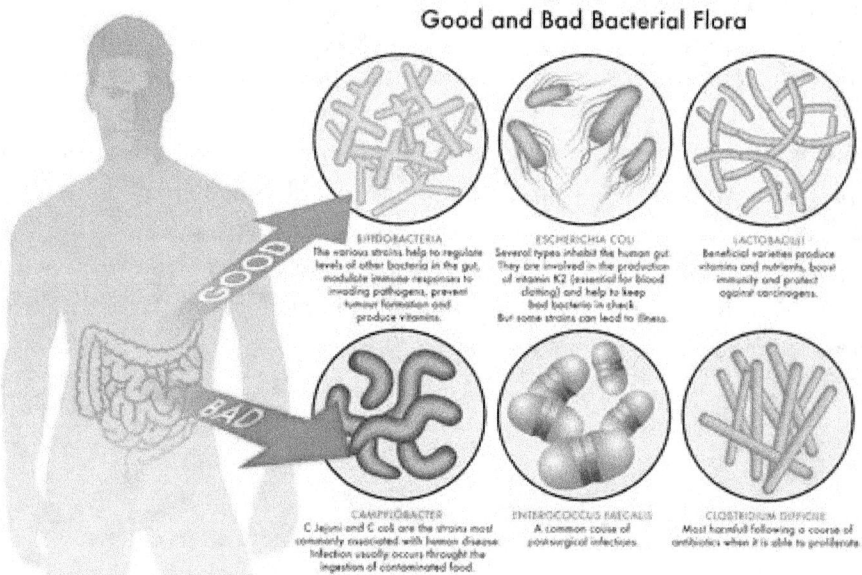

Lactobacillus:

Lactobacillus is a kind of bacteria than can be divided again into 50 more species; there are naturally found in the urinary, digestive and genital systems. They can be incorporated into the body by consuming fermented foods like yogurt or dietary supplements. Lactobacillus has been in use for treating a wide array of diseases in the human body.

One of the most well-known types of Lactobacillus is Lactobacillus GG which, when given to children between the ages of 5 and 14 suffering from irritable bowel syndrome, reduced the frequency as well as severity of abdominal pain. The dose given to these children were 3 billion cells, twice a day. Lactobacillus GG was given to children taking antibiotics and it was found that there was a decrease in the number of cases of diarrhea that came out. Traveler's diarrhea was also reduced by the intake of Lactobacillus GG. It was found out that the risk decreased by 47% in 245 people travelling in 14 different regions. Moreover, Lactobacillus GG milk was able to decrease the occurrence as well as severity of lung infections in children between the ages of 1 and 6.

Bifidobacteria:

When it comes to this particular genus, it has approximately 30 species and makes up most of the healthy bacteria in our colon. They are known to have a significantly high presence in the intestinal tract right from the days of birth, notably in breastfed infants.

Species most commonly used as probiotics include Bifidobacteria bifidum, Bifidobacteria longum, Bifidobacteria lactis, Bifidobacteria brevem, Bifidobacteria thermophilum, and Bifidobacteria infantis.

Bifidobacteria have shown to be effective against dental cavities, glucose intolerance, and reduced blood lipid levels.

- In a study encompassing patients with irritable bowel syndrome, Bifidobacteria infantis was shown to improve the symptoms of abdominal pain, bowel dysfunction, bloating, straining and incomplete evacuation of gas.

- Bifidobacteria lactis has been reported to have beneficial effects on the metabolism like lowering bad cholesterol in type-2 diabetics, increased levels of good cholesterol and glucose tolerance.

Others:

Saccharomyces boulardii is a bacterium known to be the only yeast probiotic; studies have shown that it is effective in treating diarrhea caused by side-effects induced by antibiotics. It has been in use to treat acne and reduce the side effects of the treatment for *Helicobacter pylori.* Streptococcus thermophilus is another type of bacterium that has been shown to produce large quantities of the enzyme lactase, making it an effective probiotic in the treatment of lactose intolerance.

Chapter # 4: Dosage

Fermented dairy products are popularly known as the biggest source of probiotics. However, there are other sources to these beneficial bacteria too; they are listed as:

- Cereals
- Juice
- Frozen Yogurt
- Granola bars & cookies
- Kefir
- Aged cheeses
- Kimchi
- Miso
- Sauerkraut
- Tempeh
- Pickles
- Kombucha tea

Yogurt:

After the pasteurization process, manufacturers tend to add active cultures of bacteria beneficial to the digestive system to the yogurt. Kefir is a cultured product produced by the addition of large amounts of healthy bacteria to milk. Yogurt and kefir are both almost equally beneficial for the body and even though the amount of bacteria in these food items is less than many supplements, people with bowel dysfunction can benefit from them.

Bacteria to look out for:

Many health-promoting strains of bacteria have been listed in the preceding chapter, however if one is looking to repopulate the digestive system with healthy bacteria, any supplement or food item taken must contain Lactobacillus acidophilus, Bifidobacteria bifidum, Lactobacillus casei and Streptococcus thermophilus.

A dose of 5-10 billion CFUs, or colony forming units, is ideal; keep in mind that as probiotics are living organisms they require certain conditions during their production, delivery and storage to remain effective. One should also not expect to gain all the benefits from an inexpensive probiotic supplement, again, due to the reasons stated earlier.

The requirements that a microbe must fulfill in order to be considered as a probiotic is that:

- It must be alive when being monitored

- It must have a health benefit

- It must be monitored at levels where it can provide these health benefits.

As mentioned earlier, when taking a probiotic supplement the conditions of storage provided by the manufacturer must be followed carefully. The other thing to remember is that not all microorganisms are created equally; the genus, strain and species must all be same as that in a study if you wish to achieve similar results.

With the ever growing popularity of probiotics, there is always a huge array of supplements you can choose from. The most important thing to keep in mind is that it's not the quantity of these bacteria that matters but the particular probiotic for a medical condition that does. In case you can't understand this, your best bet is visiting your doctor and taking his/her advice regarding both the type and quantity of probiotic supplements you should take.

Health Benefits

Chapter # 1: Diarrhea

Diarrhea is a digestive disorder that involves the passing of loose or watery stools after small intervals of time; it is the direct opposite of constipation and can have causes that can be both infectious as well as non-infectious. About 30 percent of the people who take antibiotics tend to suffer from diarrhea and the reason behind this is simple: antibiotics that are originally designed to take on disease causing bacteria also have a negative impact on healthy intestinal flora; this results in patients suffering from diarrhea and other gastrointestinal distresses. Probiotics can alleviate the symptoms of diarrhea if taken before and during an antibiotic dose. Lactobacillus GG and Saccharomyces boulardii have shown the greatest amount of effectiveness with respect to this problem.

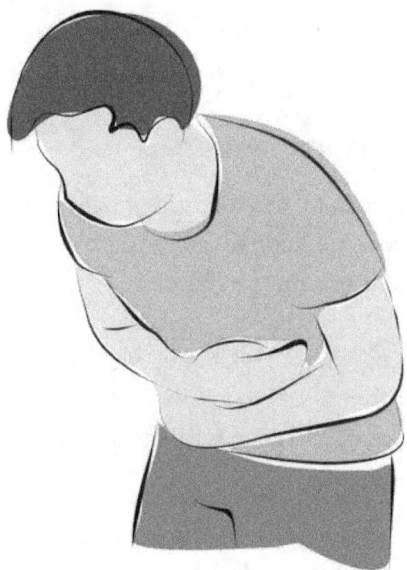

Probiotic therapy has shown some of its best results in the treatment of diarrhea. Controlled trials have shown that Lactobacillus GG has the ability to shorten the time frame of the infectious diarrhea in both infants and children, but not adults. This report was significantly important because diarrhea proves fatal mostly in children due to their lack of sustenance to dehydration. For this particular study 81 children, between the age of 1 and 3, who were hospitalized for reasons not including diarrhea, were chosen in a randomly assigned trial to test the effectiveness of Lactobacillus GG. 45 children were given a 6x10 dose of the probiotic while 36 were kept on a placebo diet. The results showed that the bacteria successfully reduced the risk of infectious diarrhea compared to placebo: 6.7% vs. 33.3% figuratively speaking. The bacteria also reduced the risk of rotavirus gastroenteritis, an infection in the digestive tract that causes fever, vomiting along with diarrhea, down to 2.2%. This successfully showed probiotics at work in the digestive tract.

Another very common variant of diarrhea is Traveler's Diarrhea that is caused by consumption of contaminated food during travelling; up to 10% of diarrhea developed while travelling ends up in persistent diarrhea. Three particular genuses of good bacteria have shown the strongest evidence in helping against this ailment:

    i.   Saccharomyces boulardii

    ii.   Lactobacillus acidophilus

    iii.   Bifidobacteria bifidum

Diarrhea can also be caused by the infectious bacteria C. difficile; in this case the diarrhea can become very severe and sometimes even life threatening. The problem becomes even more severe with repeat infections of the bacterium that make it very difficult to control. In a large study, patients with recurrent episodes of diarrhea were given the probiotics Saccharomyces boulardii and Lactobacillus GG; it was found that only 9 out of 26 patients had further recurrence while those on the placebo treatment had 22 events of recurrent out of 34.

It can be seen that Saccharomyces boulardii is being used again and again in the treatment of different types of diarrhea. In fact, the probiotic has proven so effective that scientists are recommending it as a remedy to:

    i.   Acute diarrhea

    ii.   Irritable Bowel Syndrome

    iii.   Inflammatory Bowel Syndrome

iv.   Crohn's Disease

v.   Recurrent Clostridium

Chapter # 2: Brain Function

Bacteria are not just limited to the digestive tract but can also affect the normal function of the brain, according to new scientific breakthroughs. It was discovered by scientists that the brain had the ability to send signals to the gut; this explains why episodes of gastrointestinal problems are often caused by stress.

A study was conducted by researchers at the University of California Los Angeles and was published in the journal *Gastroenterology*, which aimed at studying the brain function of healthy women who consumed probiotic yogurt. A total of 36 women, who were between the ages of 18 – 55 were chosen for this study and split into 3 groups:

- The first group was given yogurt containing a mix of several probiotics, twice daily for four weeks.

- The second group was given a dairy product with no probiotic.

- The third group was kept on no special diet.

The function of the women's brain changed while they were in resting state and in the middle of emotion-recognition tasks. In order to have greater insight, the researchers carried out functional magnetic resonance imaging on each patient's brain, before and after the study period. The emotion-recognition tasks included making the women look at angry & frightened faces; these were performed to judge the cognitive brain regions' reaction to visual stimulus. It was found out that during these tasks, the first group experienced less activity in both areas of the cortex that are known to process internal body sensations. Furthermore, the women who consumed the probiotic yogurt had decreased activity in the emotional, sensory and cognitive regions of the brain, compared to the two other groups. In the resting state there was greater connection between the two regions responsible for increased cognitive effectiveness.

This new discovery of the connection between the gut and the brain lead the associate professor Dr. Kirsten Tillisch, who was also the lead author, to conclude that yogurt may actually change the way the brain reacts to a particular event. The researchers are now focusing on finding the chemicals in the gut that caused these signals to be sent to the brain. In addition, the researchers hope to find out a relation between intestinal content and cure to diseases like Alzheimer's and Parkinson's.

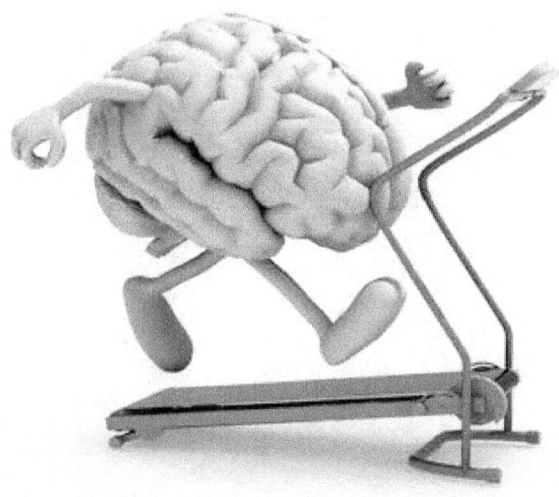

Another extremely valuable breakthrough into the linkage between the brain and intestinal tract was made by researchers from the Alimentary Pharmobiotic Centre at the University College Cork and Brain-Body Institute at McMaster University Canada. The research showed that probiotics had the potential to alter the brain's neurochemistry to treat depression & anxiety related disorders. The study was carried out using the probiotic Lactobacillus rhamnosus and was carried out on mice. The results of the study showed that mice that were just fed with broth had fewer anxiety and depression-related cases. Moreover, the bacteria also caused a decrease in the levels of a stress-induced hormone, corticosterone. The results also showed that when the mice were regularly fed with Lactobacillus rhamnosus, the receptors for a neurotransmitter in the mouse's brain were altered. This was the first time any direct impact of probiotics had been seen on the brain. With this, it was established that the vagus nerve was responsible for the gut-brain communication and therefore, probiotics having an impact in this region would prove to be the most effective against cognitive diseases.

Chapter # 3: Cholesterol

What is cholesterol? The answer is simple but not easy; cholesterol is both a friend and an enemy. It is an essential substance required for the body's normal functioning but if the levels get too high, it becomes a danger to the whole cardiovascular system. There are two types of cholesterol:

i. LDL cholesterol or bad cholesterol

ii. HDL cholesterol or good cholesterol

Probiotics have drawn an unprecedented amount of attention towards themselves due to their seemingly unlimited uses and scientists have found out that lowering LDL cholesterol is one of them. A study presented in the American Heart Association's Scientific Sessions 2012 concluded that two daily doses of probiotics can lead to lower levels of bad and total cholesterol in the body. Researchers studied the effect of the probiotic Lactobacillus Reuteri in lowering LDL and the cholesterol molecules attached to fatty acids; this cholesterol molecule-fatty acid combination accounts for the greatest amount of blood cholesterol that leads to cardiovascular disease.

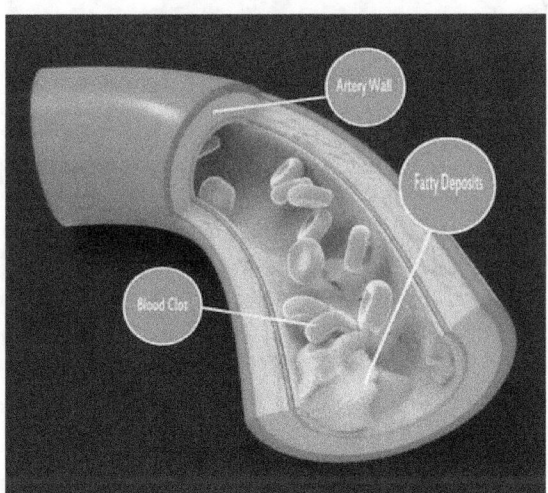

The study involved around 127 patients with high cholesterol, all of whom were adults. Half the participants were given the probiotic twice a day while the rest were kept on placebo diet. After nine weeks, those on the probiotic had LDL levels 11.6 % lower than the other group. Also the cholesterol esters were reduced by 6.3% and ester-fatty acid combination by 8.3%. The total cholesterol in the probiotic group decreased by 9.1%, while the levels of blood triglycerides and HDL cholesterol remained unchanged. The researchers proposed that the bacteria Lactobacillus Reuteri was singlehandedly responsible for lowering the levels of cholesterol along with breaking apart molecules known as bile salts. The researchers linked the breakup of bile salts with levels of LDL cholesterol by measuring the levels of both substances; it was found that breakup of bile salts lead to reduced cholesterol absorption in the gut and thus a reduced level of LDL cholesterol.

The probiotic was given in doses of 200 mg a day, far lower than other treatments used against high levels of cholesterol.

Chapter # 4: Infections

Infection is the invasion and replication of microorganisms such as bacteria and viruses, not normally present in the body. An infection can be with or without symptoms and can remain localized or spread throughout the body using the blood and become systemic.

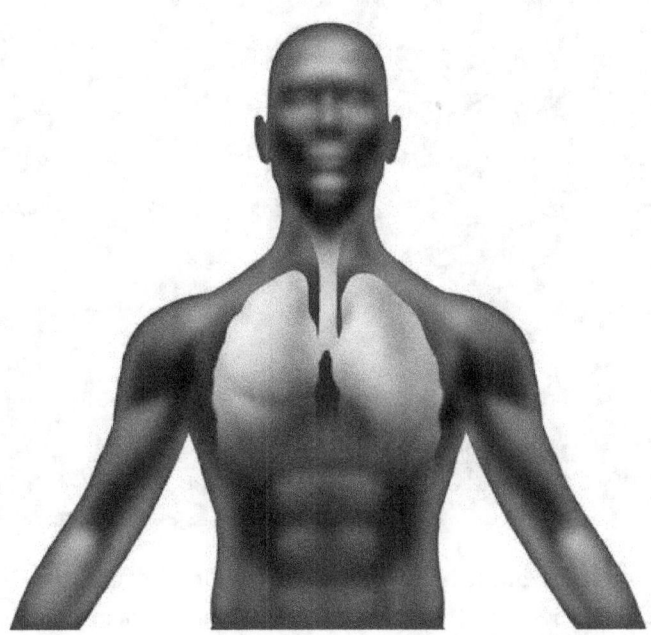

Scientists at University College Cork have discovered that probiotics can deliver against infections caused by bacteria. The discovery took place in the Alimentary Pharmobiotic Centre in UCC and was published in *Proceedings of the National Academy of Sciences*. The group examined the effects of a number of beneficial bacteria and found that one particular probiotic, Lactobacillus salivarius, was able to kill the lethal pathogens, Listeria monocytogenes, found in pregnant women. The probiotic achieved this feat by creating a compound similar to an antibiotic known as bacteriocin. It was further found out that it was only Lactobacillus salivarius that offered protection against the pathogen and no other strain of the same genus was able to achieve the same amount of protection. The results are quite significant as Listeria monocytogenes are very dangerous during pregnancy and is too rare for a full-scale vaccination to take place. Therefore, a probiotic taken during pregnancy can provide the best protection against this pathogen that otherwise might prove hazardous.

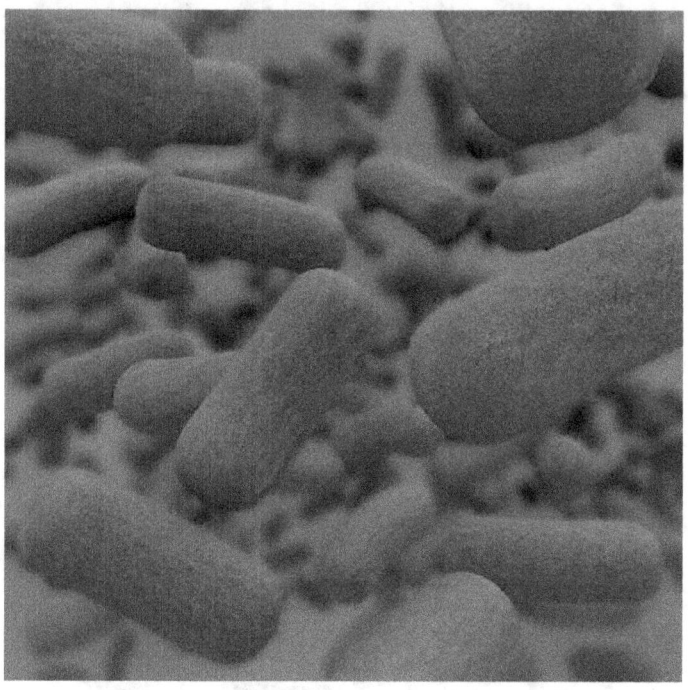

According to a study published in the British Journal of Sports Medicine, long distance runners who took probiotics had shorter, as well as, less intense spells of illness than runners on placebo treatment. The researchers stated that endurance athletes who went through rugged training were heavily open to upper respiratory tract infections; exercise could leave the immunity system unchecked, leaving the athletes vulnerable to viruses that could cause coughs, cold and flu. The participants of the study consisted of 20 elite athletes who were going through four months of winter training. The athletes were each given either three frozen capsules, twice a day of the probiotic Lactobacillus fermentum or a dummy capsule. The supplement was administered over a period of 28 days followed by a month long hiatus which was again followed by a 28 day administration of the body. This allowed the athletes to take the probiotic for a month without any external effects influencing the results. During the study, the researchers analyzed the treadmill performance, immune response and the severity plus length of respiratory tract infections. During the probiotic treatment period, about half as many upper respiratory tract infections along with lower respiratory illness events were reported when compared with the placebo time period. Even though the length of each event didn't differ between the placebo and probiotic groups, the total number of days of illness differed significantly; just 30 days compared to 72 days for the placebo group. Furthermore, the severity of symptoms was also milder with the probiotic group that lead to no change in running performance compared to the placebo group.

Many women treat recurring yeast infections by eating or sometimes inserting yogurt into the vaginal area; this is widely considered a folk remedy and is backed by limited medical science support but nonetheless is practically implemented by many.

Chapter # 5: Chronic Fatigue & Psoriasis

Psoriasis is a long term, non-contagious skin problem that causes the skin cells to grow swiftly, resulting in white, silvery or red, thick patches of skin. Normally, new skin cells replace the old ones as the outer layers of the skin are shed but in psoriasis, the new skin cells move to the surface in days, rather than weeks, resulting in buildup of thick patches called plaques. It is a common ailment in adults but can also occur in adolescents too.

Chronic fatigue syndrome is a sophisticated disorder that is characterized by episodes of extreme fatigue that can't be reasoned by an underlying medical condition. The fatigue can worsen with mental or physical activity but does not improve with rest. The cause of the syndrome is unknown and ranges from viral infections to mental stress.

Scientists from Alimentary Health & Alimentary Pharmobiotic Centre at University College Cork have shown that a probiotic, commercially available in the US, previously known for its gastrointestinal benefits, has the ability to treat non-gut inflammations, as well as, chronic fatigue syndrome and psoriasis. The study is the first one to show that microbes have benefits outside the mucosal immune system. The mucosal immune system is responsible for the protection of internal tracts such as gastrointestinal, respiratory and urogenital ones. These tracts act as barriers to the outside world for the internal tissues of the body that are then again protected by a layer known as the systematic immune system.

For the study, the gut friendly probiotic Bifidobacteria infantis was used; three separate placebo-controlled trials were performed to study the effect of the bacterium on gastrointestinal and non-gastrointestinal disorders. Firstly, 22 patients with the gastrointestinal disorder, ulcerative colitis were recruited, then 48 patients with chronic fatigue syndrome were recruited and finally 35 healthy volunteers were chosen to act as reference point for the levels of inflammation in patients that went on trial. A total of three biomarkers were used in the study that included C-reactive protein, pro-inflammatory cytokines, interleukin-6 and tumor necrosis alpha. The trial period lasted between 6 to 8 weeks, during which both the patients and the healthy volunteers were given sachets containing either the probiotic or a dummy medicine.

At the start of the trial it was found that each patient had significantly raised levels of the 3 biomarkers of inflammation compared to the healthy volunteers. However at the end:

- All of the 3 groups who received the probiotic supplement had lower levels of CRP.

- The patients suffering from CFS and psoriasis showed reduction in the TNF-a.

- The patients suffering from UC and CFS showed reductions in IL-6.

These results showed that probiotics were at work in reducing symptoms of inflammation in the body.

Recipes

Chapter # 1: Fermented Hot Chili Sauce

Makes: About a quart

Prep time: 20 minutes

Cooking time: 5 to 7 days (fermentation)

Ingredients:

- 3 pounds of fresh chili peppers (Jalapenos, Scotch bonnets, Serrano, etc)

- 2 tablespoons unrefined cane sugar

- 4 to 6 cloves of garlic, peeled and minced

- 2 teaspoons of unrefined sea salt

- Vegetable starter culture in ¼ cup water, dissolved

Directions:

First, snip the stems from the chilies, leaving the green tops intact. Combine all the ingredients in a food processor, or mince by hand until it a fine texture is achieved. Next, spoon the chili paste in a glass mason jar and cover it at room temperature for five to seven days so it can ferment properly. After the chili paste has bubbled for about a week, set a fine mesh sieve on a mixing bowl and spoon the chili paste out. With a wooden spoon, press the paste into the side of the sieve so that the sauce drips from the sieve into the mixing bowl. Once you've pressed the chili sauce, pour it from the mixing bowl to a jar or bottle and store it in a refrigerator; this will ensure its maximum freshness for days to come.

Chapter # 2: Probiotic Apple & Beetroot Relish

Makes: Approximately 24, 2 ounce portions

Prep time: 10 – 20 minutes

Cooking time: 3 – 4 days

Ingredients:

1. 3 large apples (1 ½ pounds)

2. 3 large beets (1 ½ pounds)

3. 2 star anise pods

4. 1 tablespoon unrefined sea salt

5. 1 tablespoon whole cloves

6. Fermented vegetable starter culture

Directions:

First, shred the apples and beets with your hands or using a food processor. Then toss the shredded items together until they are well combined. Add the star anise and cloves to the mixture and continue to toss the whole thing until the spices are distributed among the fruits & vegetables. Next, in a vegetable fermenter, layer the apple and beetroot and intermittently sprinkle unrefined sea salt over the layers of fruits & veggies. Then mash them with a mallet to encourage the items giving up their juices. After this, ferment in a vegetable fermenter for a period of 3 to 4 days; more time may be required depending on the warmth of your kitchen. After the given time period, remove the apple & beetroot relish from the fermenter and pick out the star anise pods plus the whole cloves. Place the mixture into a blender and process it until it turns smooth.

Chapter # 3: Moroccan Preserved Lemons

Makes: ½ gallon

Prep time: 10 minutes

Ingredients:

1. 2 ½ pounds lemons

2. ¼ cup unrefined sea salt

Directions:

Trim the ends off lemons, making sure not to cut into the flesh of any of them. Slice the lemons into quarters, and keep the base intact. Sprinkle the interiors of the lemons with the sea salt and then layer them in a fermentation device. Spoon, until the rinds of the lemon begin to soften and the lemons release their juices. Continue mashing, salting and repeating the process again until the lemons successfully fill the jar by elevating above the juice. Finally, ferment at room temperature for 3 – 4 weeks and you have yourself Moroccan lemons good for a whole year.

Conclusion

There's a battle going on in the intestinal tract, and the bacteria outnumber the cells 10 to 1; fortunately not all these bacteria are bad and in fact there are many good bacteria currently making sure that your body doesn't fall prey to the bad ones. The good bacteria, also known as probiotics, have been in use for thousands of years in the form of dairy products, vegetables, etc. However, scientists have just discovered these health-promoting microbes and have been astounded by their beneficial properties. Many of these bacteria are already present in the body and you just need to boost up your reserves whenever you go on medication or suffer from a specific disease. Which probiotic to take and when to take; these and all other questions have been answered in this book and it would be a shame if you don't use them to your advantage.

References

1. http://www.fotolia.com/id/45257208

2. http://www.fotolia.com/id/48980656

3. http://www.fotolia.com/id/45156048

4. http://www.fotolia.com/id/53256130

5. http://www.fotolia.com/id/38713127

6. http://www.123rf.com/photo_26101438_probiotics-red-rubber-stamp-over-a-white-background.html

7. http://www.123rf.com/photo_29466432_stock-vector-intestinal-bacterial-flora.html

8. http://www.123rf.com/photo_6729187_3d-illustration-of-a-colony-of-bacteria-with-depth-of-field.html?term=probiotic

9. http://www.123rf.com/photo_11242506_stomach-ache.html?term=diarrhea

10. http://www.123rf.com/photo_11359781_cold-flu-cough-sinus-and-congestion-symptoms-medical-health-symbol-with-a-human-and-lungs-congested-.html?term=infection

Author Bio

Muhammad Usman is a distinguished medical graduate of Allama iqbal medical college (AIMC). He is a professional writer who has been in the field for more than 4 years. During this time he has produced 10,000+ articles, blogs and eBooks on various niches related to diseases, health, fitness, nutrition and well-being. He is a regular contributor to several journals related to medicine and surgery. He is the editor of several journals and newspapers.

Check out some of the other JD-Biz Publishing books

Gardening Series on Amazon

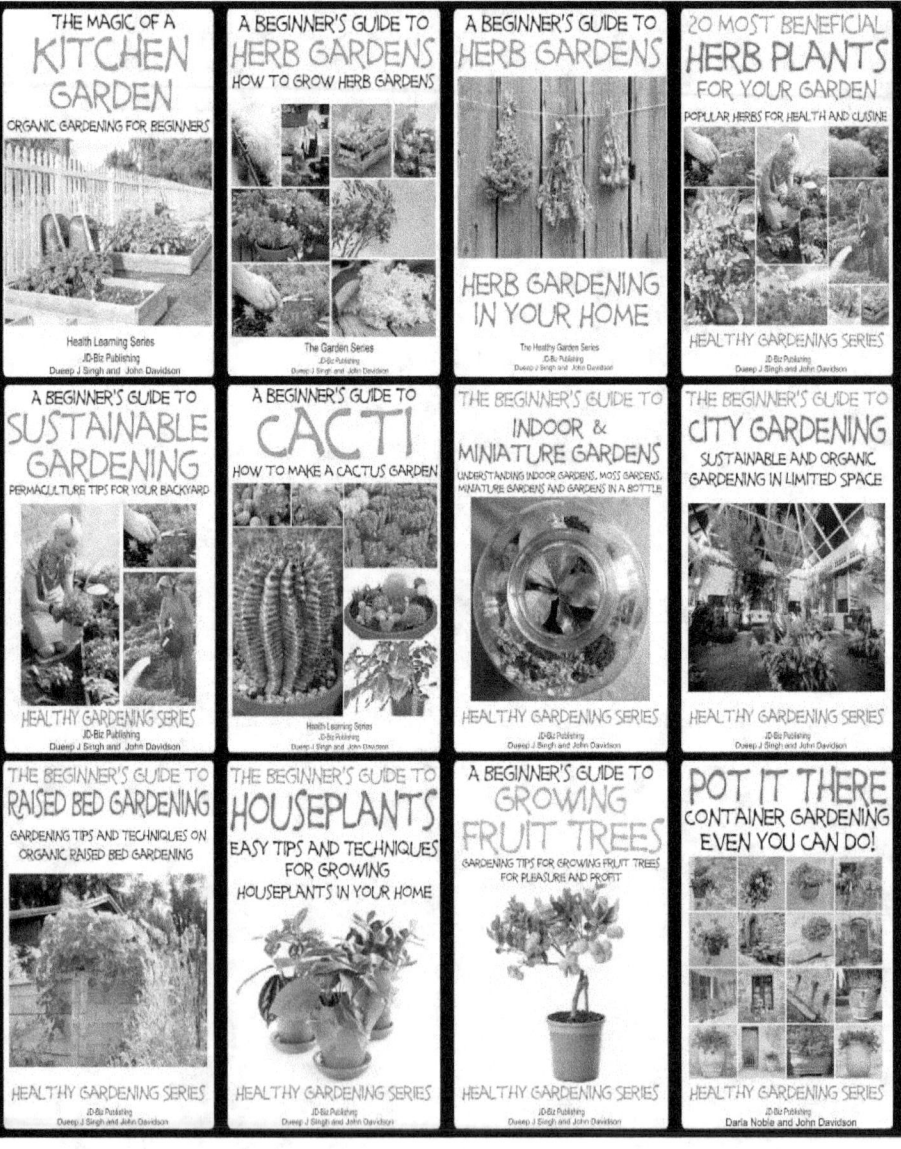

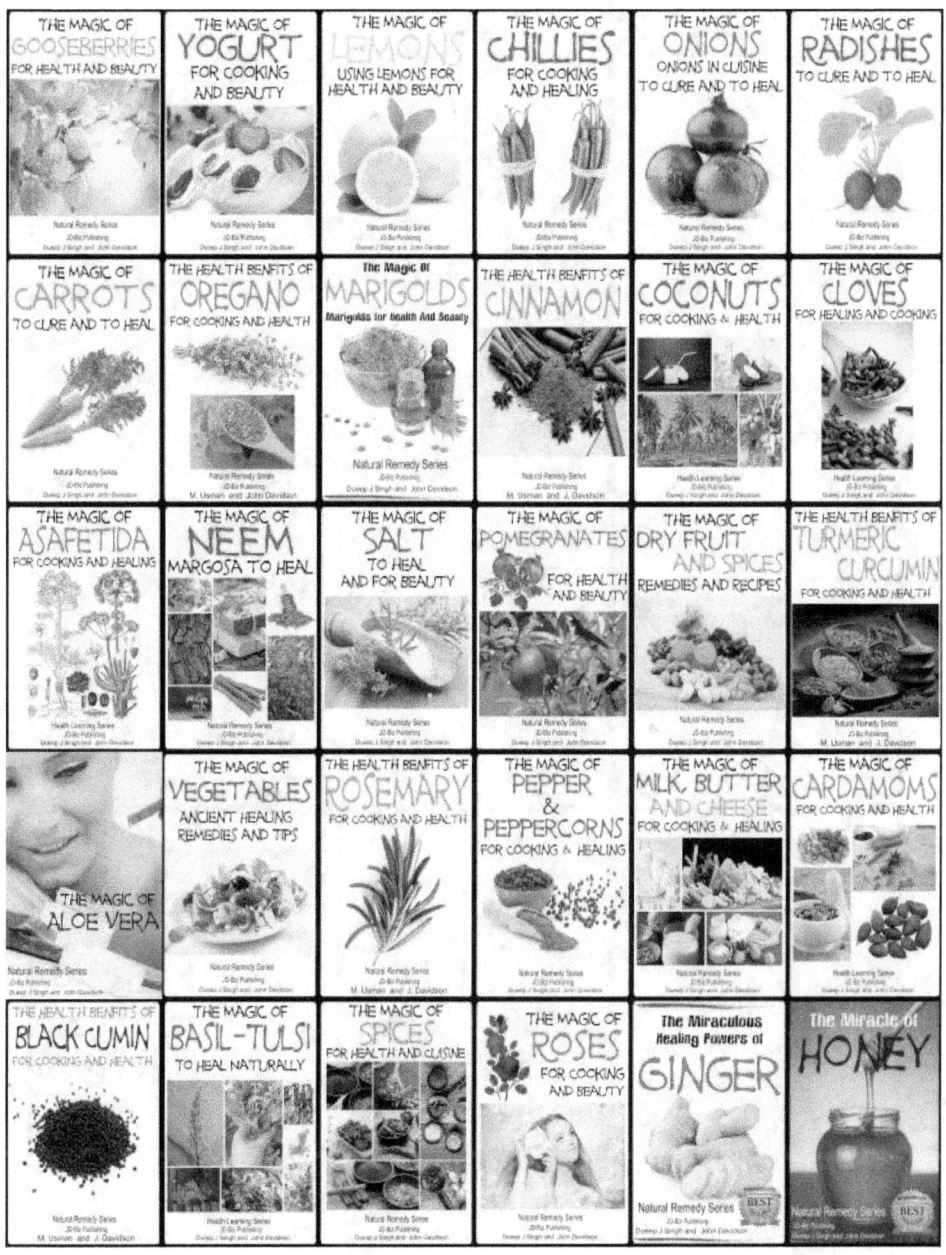

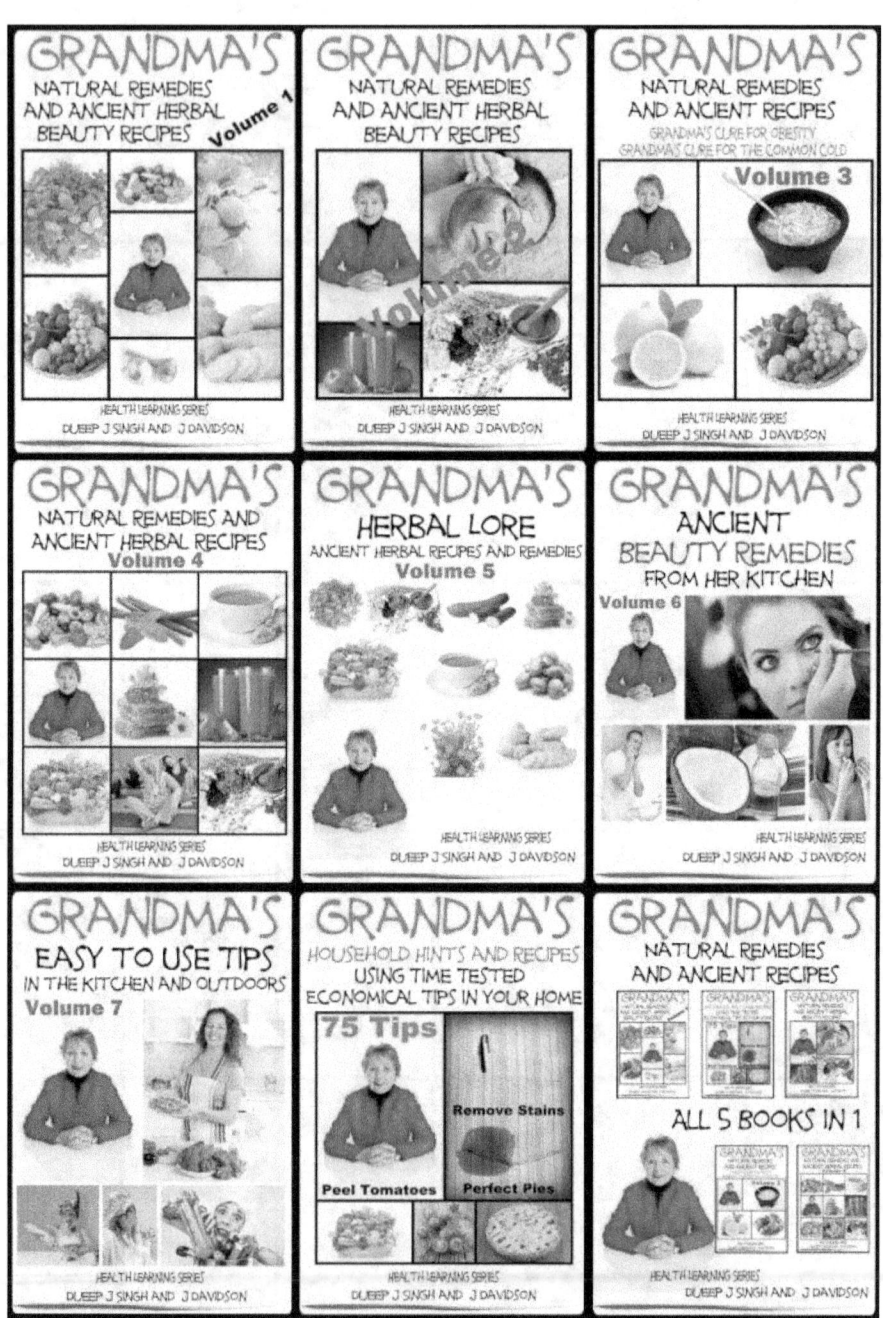

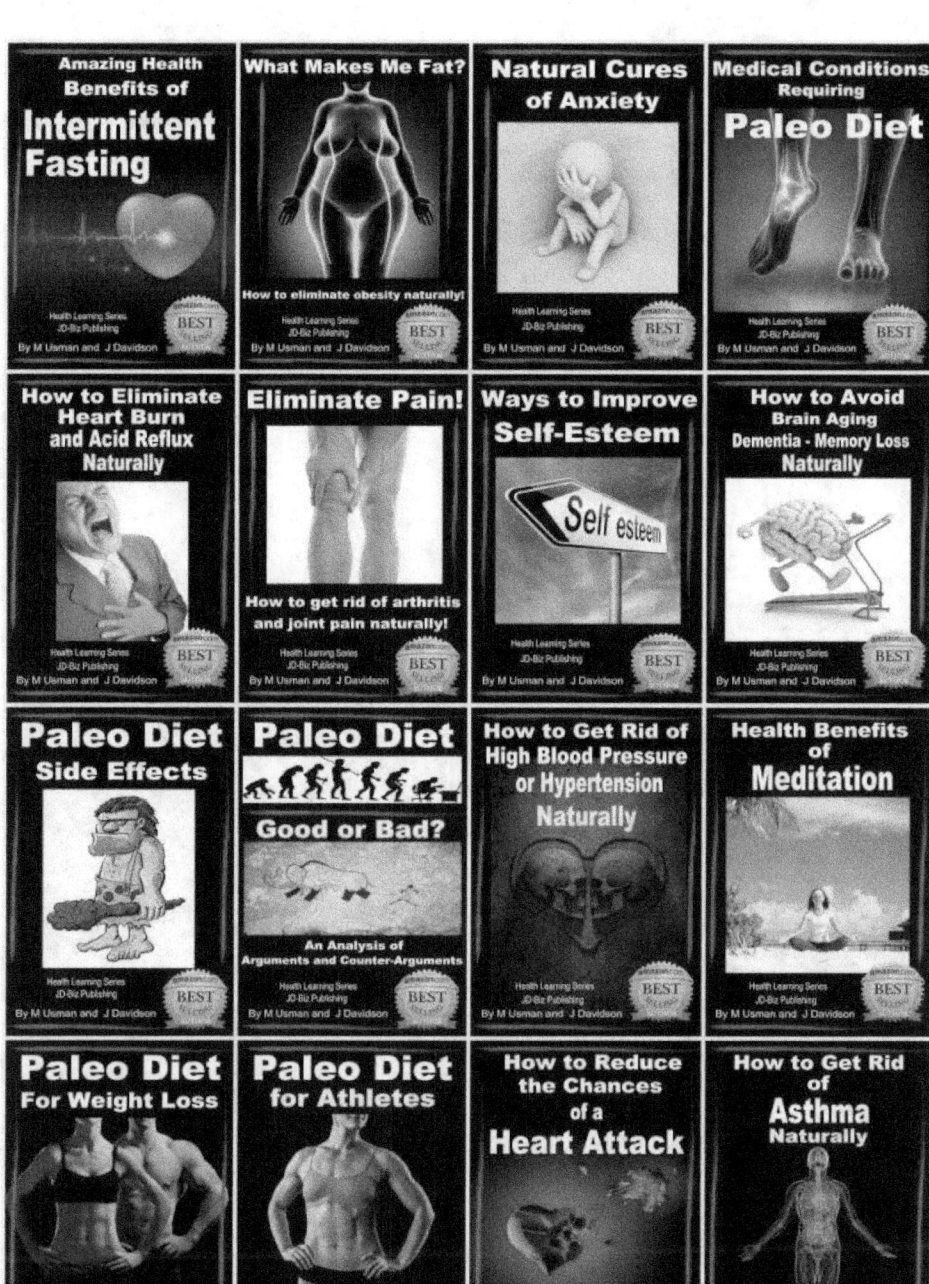

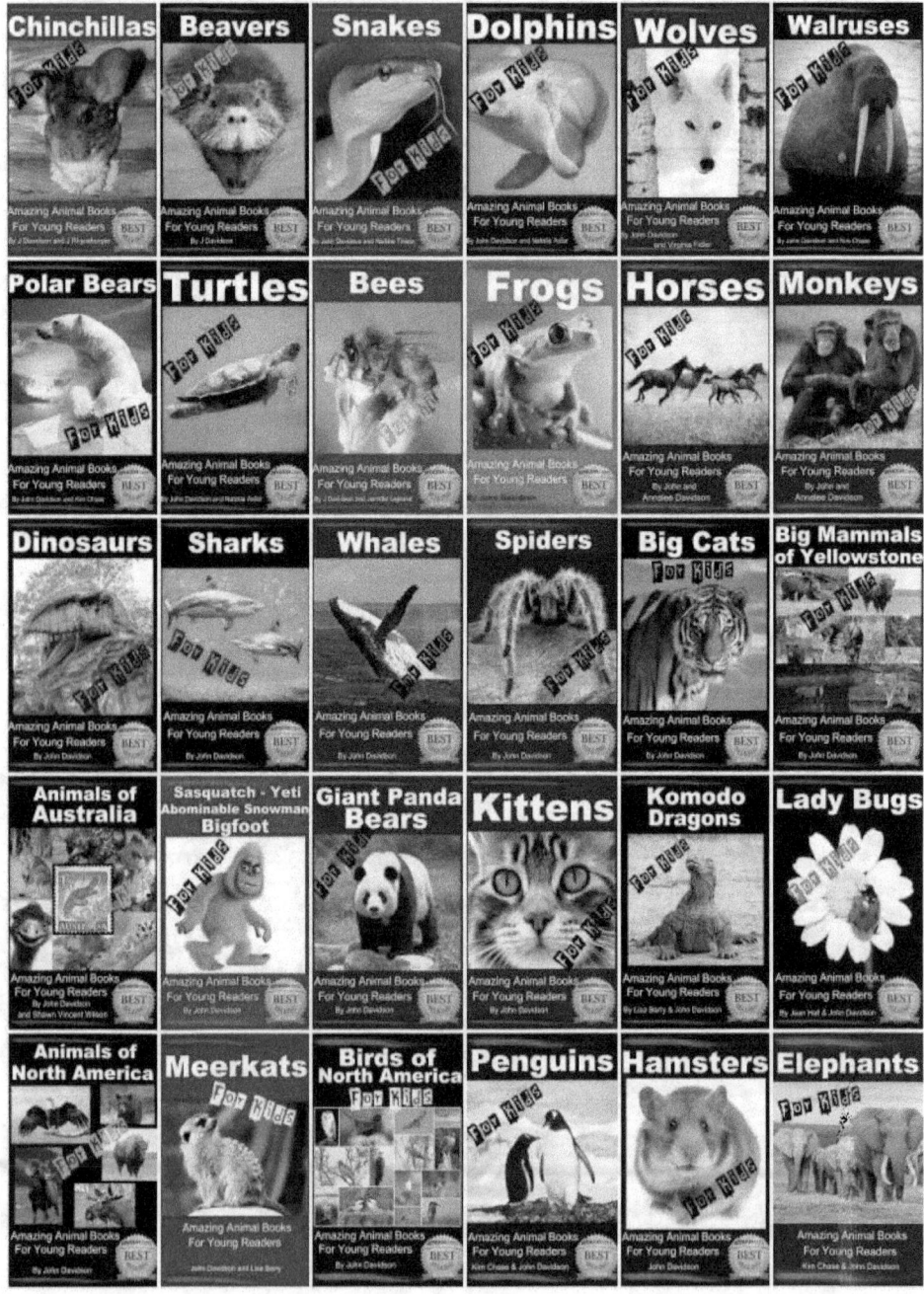

Learn To Draw Series

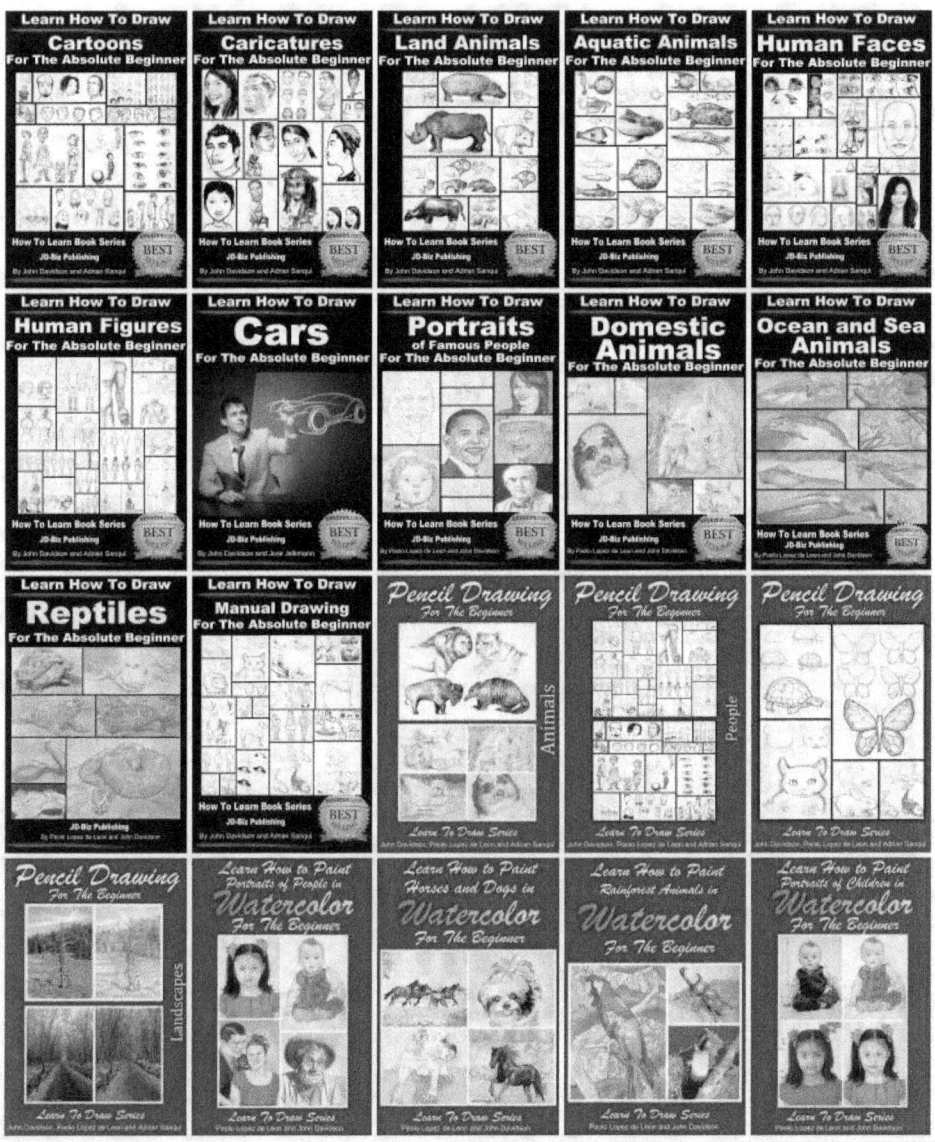

How to Build and Plan Books

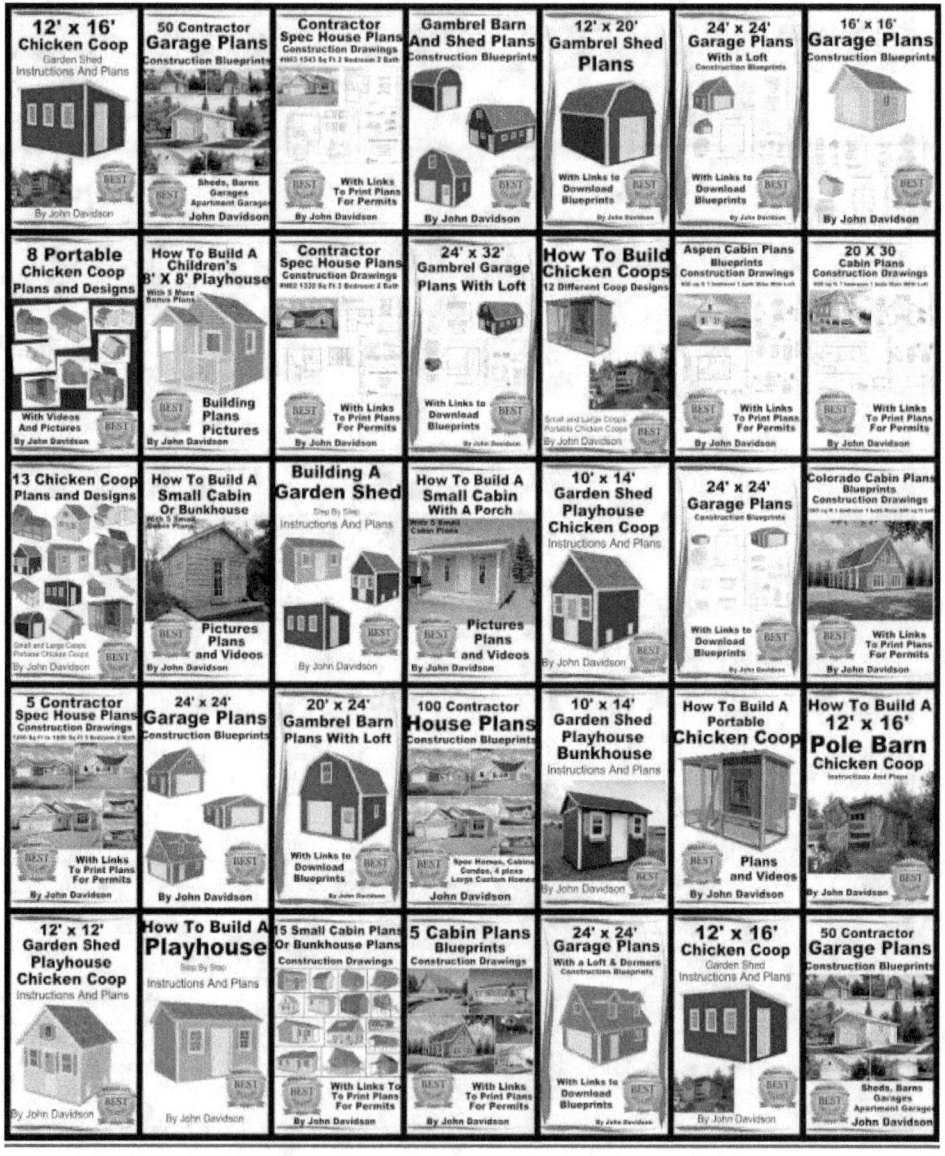

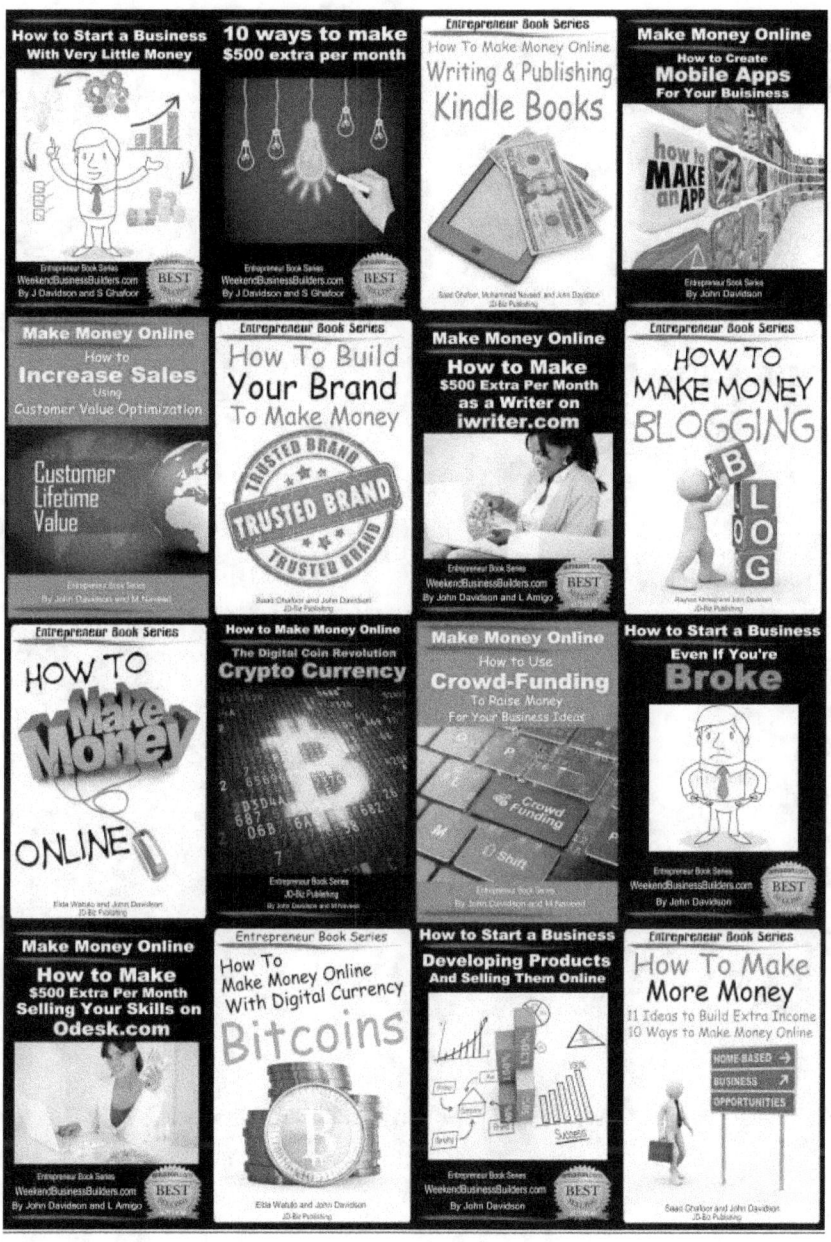

Our books are available at

1. Amazon.com

2. Barnes and Noble

3. Itunes

4. Kobo

5. Smashwords

6. Google Play Books

This book is published by

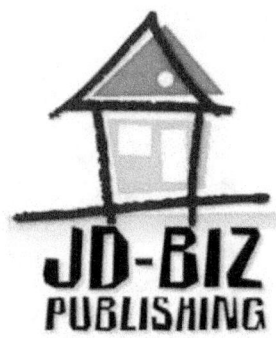

JD-Biz Corp

P O Box 374

Mendon, Utah 84325

http://www.jd-biz.com/

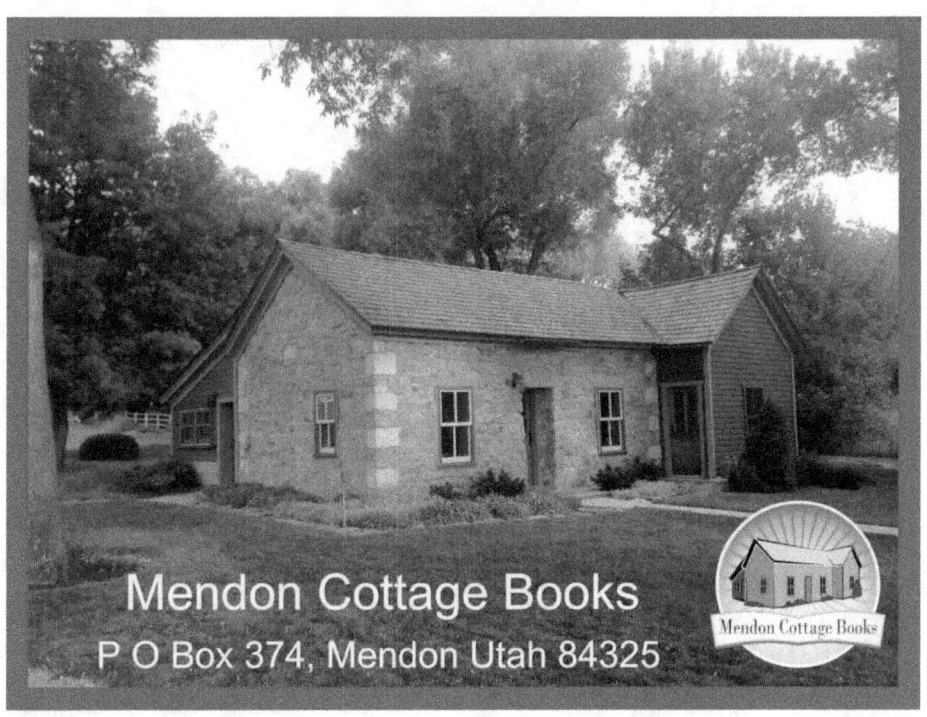

Mendon Cottage Books

P O Box 374, Mendon Utah 84325

www.ingramcontent.com/pod-product-compliance
Lightning Source LLC
Chambersburg PA
CBHW061927280526
45787CB00004B/1515

* 9 781505 574715 *